The Real Guide to Gluten

lauren r. hatfield

ISBN-13: 978-1506129006
ISBN-10: 1506129005

Disclaimer: Please seek medical advice from a licensed professional prior to making any changes in your diet or exercise routine. I am not a doctor, though much of my research over the years has come from skilled medical professionals and literature written by experts in medicine. My tips and tricks may not apply to everyone, as each case is unique, but I strive to give you accurate and helpful information as you're embarking on this journey.

dedication

This book was written to encourage all who have endured the labyrinth of chronic GI illness - especially those who have not been successful with a diagnosis or treatment. My prayer is that this personal story will be a blessing to others going through their own difficult journey.

contents

acknowledgments

introduction 1

my tale 7

the basics 21

- gluten guide & cheat sheets 22
- celiac disease symptoms 25

pregnancy, parenting, & gluten 27

- pregnancy & gluten 28
- labor & delivery 32
- breastfeeding & first foods 35
- gf parenting 37
- gluten cheat sheet for teachers, coaches, etc. 40

the 'hit' list 47

gf chef 59

appetizers 63

main dishes 69

side dishes 85

desserts 99

coming out of the pantry 111

acknowledgements

Everything I do is for the honor and glory of my precious Savior. 1 Corinthians 10:31

introduction

There you sit on the sofa, destroying a bottle of wine, and wondering what in the world went wrong. You always took care of yourself and ate healthy. Well, mostly. Ok, some of the time. Fine, a girl can't resist chocolate and cheesecake here and there. But overall, you've made wise choices. I mean, come on, when you look at those around you, you're doing great! You were minding your own business when that jerk doctor had to screw it all up. He handed you the diagnosis that would change your life forever.

"I'm sorry to tell you that you have celiac disease."

For some of you, it's just gluten sensitivity (and yes, I do believe in such a thing), or perhaps a wheat allergy. For others still, you made the harrowing discovery on your own, via trial and error. Either way, the blow hits like a freight train.

Your first thoughts: "What in the world is gluten? Which medicine do we prescribe to get rid of it?" As he goes on to deliver the news that you will be 'treating' this affliction every day for the rest of your life, waving a permanent goodbye to all your favorite foods, your head starts to spin. "What about Thanksgiving…and mom's famous stuffing? What about the pasta dish I spent 8 years perfecting? What about birthday cakes and holiday goodies? What about fresh baked bread, straight from the oven? What about gooey brownies that probably should've cooked longer but I just couldn't wait to cover in ice cream and devour? What about pancakes, waffles, and cereal? What about my favorite restaurant where I begin with mouth-watering rolls and a bruschetta appetizer, followed by an entrée of chicken alfredo, and then complete with a decadent tiramisu?" A piercing crack in the universe renders you temporarily deaf as you stare blankly toward the man who delivered your sentence.

You then walk numbly out of the building, hands full of brochures for gluten free living and specialized dieticians, wondering if you would've been better off calling in sick from your doctor appointment. At least if you didn't know about it, you wouldn't have to change your entire life…forever. Right?

You snap back to your pity party, thump the bottle of wine onto the coffee table, and wander into your kitchen. You then open every last cabinet door until the room looks like a scene from Paranormal Activity, and proceed with a frantic purging of everything in sight. Beginning with the cereal cabinet, you read each label and fling whatever doesn't fit your newly imposed diet. Realizing the space is now completely empty and nothing passed the test, you move on to the next door, hoping for better results. You toss the toaster pastries over your shoulder...then the box of macaroni and cheese... the gourmet crackers you JUST spent $10 on... your stash of flour and baking supplies.... granola bars... Hamburger Helper... and the list goes on.

Suddenly, you find yourself dejected, sitting in a pile of boxes on the floor while your open cabinets reveal nothing more than cobwebs and a jar of unopened pickles. After a few moments staring aimlessly at the train wreck around you, hair a mess, you realize you need to go back to wherever you left the wine.

I feel your pain. Ok, perhaps it was slightly less dramatic for some of you, but in your own way, this revelation changed your life forever.

As a girl who lived through the diagnosis just after my college years (when I should've been more concerned with packing on the "freshman fifteen"), I can identify with the struggles you've probably encountered. In fact, at that time, there was much less awareness about the condition, as well as less alternative products available on the market. Throughout my years with the illness, I have read seemingly every book, every blog, every 'helpful' website, every do/don't list, and every brochure that friends and doctors suggest. Whether I liked it or not, it became a part of my identity. Anytime a friend saw the words 'gluten' or 'celiac,' they immediately thought of me or sent me whatever they found, hoping it would be helpful or my miracle cure. Though I knew their intentions were altruistic, I grew exhausted of the way this condition began to define me. I also became weary of everyone having the answers to a condition they hadn't endured. And worst of all, the pile of books that guaranteed the best information on the topic were overwhelming and unrelatable.

At the end of the day, the biggest impact this change has on your life is in the psychological realm. People don't realize how much our emotion and well-being is tied to food, until it is ripped out of our hands forever. Sure, they get the concept of how we tie emotions to a comfort food or how depressing a weight loss diet can be, but when you find out this change isn't temporary, it really wears on your psyche.

Don't worry, you aren't alone. The phrase may say not to cry over spilled milk, but I give you full permission to cry your heart out over spilled wheat. Or, for those of you who are also lactose intolerant like me, go ahead and cry over the milk, too.

Therefore, my gift to you is this collection of tips, tricks, and a few practical recipes from a girl who has also weathered the storm. As they say, "misery loves company;" and while I won't disillusion you to believe that all the struggles disappear, I will commiserate with you and show you some ways to make it a lot easier, along with the input of some others walking the same journey.

It's tough when no one else gets it, so let me be your best gluten girlfriend! Raise your glasses (or bottles, if you're the person I described earlier), and let's toast to being girls who are too fabulous to let a couple little grains get the better of us.

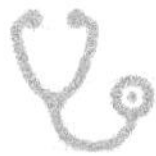

my tale

I'll try my best to be brief, but hopefully this background will show you that you aren't alone! I'm here to suffer right along with you, with hopes that my story can make you feel a little better about yours. It isn't as bubbly and refreshing a read as the rest of the book, but hopefully my struggle will help you be thankful for yours.

It all began one dark and stormy night…

Ok, perhaps not so dramatic. It was a sunny weekday, though the ominous clouds rolled in quickly. I was visiting the doctor for a routine visit in 2007, when I was asked (per the usual) if there were any concerns or strange things I've noticed going on. Usually, my answer was an energetic 'no,' but this particular visit, I happened to mention that I would get a little nauseous after eating most meals. The symptom had actually been so mild that I almost neglected to even bring it up, and it hadn't been anything that was burdening me, even in the mildest use of the word.

The doctor then asked if I noticed the symptoms with one food type more than another, which I hadn't. She then asked if I had ever heard of celiac disease. With another 'no,' she gave me a brief description, summing up gluten and how it can affect the body of someone with the condition. As a precautionary measure, she went ahead and drew my blood to test for antibodies. Couldn't hurt, right? Hmph.

I went home without giving it another thought until later in the evening. I was sitting on the sofa when that conversation returned to me, and I decided to do a little research on the condition. I was convinced I had nothing to worry about, and that my otherwise flawless health past would hold to its good name. However, always eager to learn something new, I researched the details of what gluten was and what sorts of food contained this component. Shocked by the answers that were revealed, I distinctly remember saying to myself, "Wow. It's in EVERYTHING. Man, I feel so bad for these people – what an awful life to live!"

I walked over to my kitchen to peek at ingredient labels, and only further pitied celiacs after realizing my cabinets were a gluten field day. Still confident that I had nothing to worry about, I slept peacefully and continued living a few more days as usual.

Then the phone rang. You know how the conversation goes; it's the same for most diagnoses. The doctor requests you come in as quickly as possible, and that they'd rather give you details in person. Knowing the very reason, my heart leapt into my throat. "Surely not."

Numb, I listened to a more detailed explanation of what celiac disease is and how my life would be changing. In shock, I said, "My symptoms hardly even existed. What if I just ignore all this, and we pretend I never entered your office? My mild queasiness is something I could easily live with, and I'll just continue life as before. Is that ok?"

She said, "I'm sorry, but if someone with celiac sprue continues eating gluten, it can cause permanent damage to the lining of their intestines, as well as posing a much higher risk of cancer at an early age. You will create irreparable damage to your body. It really isn't an option at this point." I stared blankly at her. "I've got some great websites I can suggest as you're getting adjusted to the new diet, and there are even some support groups here in town that will be a fantastic resource for you."

My whole world shattered to the floor. I had always been so healthy.

Fast-forward to the story of the girl I presented in the introduction. Subtract the bottle of wine, and that was exactly what happened the night of my diagnosis. I purged every last cabinet of its gluten until I realized I had no food left.

Little by little, I grew more adjusted to the diet. I was

learning how hard it was to dine out with friends. I longingly watched while they ate my favorite foods and I munched on lettuce. Even peanut butter & jelly sandwiches or cheese & crackers gained a sparkling appeal they never held in days prior. I could no longer run out for a quick lunch, as most restaurants had no gluten free options…other than salads. And let's face it, salads for every meal get old REALLY quickly. I got to the point that if one more naïve server suggested a salad to me, I was going to shove those cherry tomatoes right up his nose.

I grew bitter, and the diet really began wearing on my psyche. I don't know what kind of iron-clad people can survive this without at least a little resulting depression, but kudos to you if you're one of them! Day after day of spending tons on gluten free foods that tasted like gritty chalk, day after day of watching friends eat the things I used to love, and holiday after holiday pining for my favorite traditional treats…caused its share of breakdowns. Even the comfort foods that once made me feel a little better when I was down became forbidden poisons.

Have you felt this way? Well, take heart, because there are four pieces of good news I can offer off the top of my head:

1. This adjustment period doesn't last forever, and eventually you learn to embrace your new lifestyle.

2. There are a LOT more options available now (versus when I was diagnosed) for better tasting

gluten free foods. There is also quite a bit more awareness among restaurants and the general public. You have more educational resources available now, too, to better prepare yourself and understand the process.

3. You get this book as an easy-to-understand cheat sheet so you can glide through the process smoothly.

4. You aren't alone! Others have walked before you, and that's part of why I'm writing this book – to show you that there are many who have felt the same way you do, and we are ready and willing to help. This will also provide shortcuts for you that took me much longer to learn in a very lonely gluten journey.

---

the journey continues

For most of you, the story has a happy ending where I left off (well, as happy as a story without cake and cookies can be, that is). Typically, if you strictly follow the diet, your body heals and you eventually feel much better on a day to day basis. You are more energetic, you have less stomach concerns, you notice a decrease in auto-immune symptoms, etc. Happy day!

As luck would have it, this was only the tip of the iceberg on my epic adventure. I was the atypical case (hey, Mom always told me that if I'm going to do something, I might as well go all out). My health began a quick decline. My symptoms grew much worse, to the point they were nearly uncontrollable (I'll spare you the sexy details).

Once my family doctor realized things were moving past her realm of expertise, she sent me to a gastroenterology specialist with Wake Forest University Baptist Medical Center. This is a name recognized throughout the country as one of the best in the medical field, and particularly in the field of digestive health. Every couple weeks, we spent ungodly amounts of money visiting the hospital for evaluations, blood tests, endoscopies, colonoscopies, hydrogen breath tests, etc. You name the test, they performed it. I felt like a lab rat, not only because of the invasive and uncomfortable testing, but also because I was running on a wheel leading nowhere.

The doctor clearly had no idea why I wasn't responding positively to a gluten free diet, but he also couldn't figure out what other mystery illness I might have that was contributing to staying so ill. The only other discovery they made was that I had recurring bacterial overgrowth (the overabundance of good bacteria found in our bodies). My system responded well to the antibiotic used to treat this condition – unfortunately, the relief only lasted a couple of days before symptoms returned.

Testing further, there was a month where I was allowed to eat anything I wanted so that the doctors could analyze how my body responded to gluten. Not only did they confirm the celiac sprue diagnosis beyond a shadow of a doubt, but the strangest thing happened: I felt better. Yes, folks, you heard right. The reintroduction of gluten to my diet made nearly all of my symptoms disappear and I felt the best I'd felt since my initial diagnosis.

As you can imagine, this only perplexed the doctors further. The experts refused to admit they had exhausted their tests and run out of ideas. Instead, they began rerunning all the tests they'd already attempted, simply because they didn't know what else to do. Each visit began with "Well, we know you have celiac disease…" Yes. We had now known that for 2 years throughout all the testing…but thanks for reminding me every couple weeks. I still had resolve left in my heart, and I refused to give up as these doctors had.

So I then went through the exhausting process of acceptance into Duke University Medical Center. With another name known worldwide for its advancements in medicine, as well as skill with complicated conditions, I was certain Duke could find an answer where others failed. It wasn't easy to get in, though. One cannot imagine how many phone minutes I burned through as I was passed around between departments; everyone insisted my case was under someone else's expertise. Once I finally found the right doctor, the process of applying and even getting the time of day from their admissions department was grueling, as well. And don't get me started on involving the insurance company.

As I endured the process, bawling from phone call to phone call, I pressed on. My weight plummeted steadily throughout all these years of illness and testing. Very little nutrition was being absorbed into my body, and I received judgmental glares/comments from those who assumed this physical state was self-inflicted. I awoke early every morning to excruciating cramping, followed by nearly 20 visits to the bathroom daily (attractive, huh?!). This made carrying on a normal life with a steady job incredibly difficult. I was so weak, exhausted, and physically ill that I spent each day going to work bearing symptoms that would've caused anyone else to call in sick. I had no choice. I also tried filing for disability, unsuccessfully.

On top of all this, I still had to eat the restricted diet, even though I didn't get any results from it (other than preventing bigger problems down the road). I knew eating the things I loved would even make me feel better, yet it was forbidden by modern medicine.

Then one day, I finally cracked my way into Duke's gastroenterology department. Elated by the success and glimmer of hope (and slightly miffed by the hour-long drive I had to make bi-weekly), I met with doctors who seemed certain they could find an answer.

More tests were performed, many of which were duplicates

from those received at Wake. They also performed a very exclusive and (at the time) cutting-edge test on my blood. This test studied my genetic predisposition to having celiac disease and the intensity with which I possessed the markers. Lucky me, I scored extremely high in all the categories – more than the doctor said he had ever encountered (I'm a SUPER CELIAC! And you thought you were cool…).

He also made further strides by discovering that I have collagenous microscopic colitis. This condition is a result of collagen build-up around the intestine, causing difficulty absorbing fluids and nutrients into the body. I was encouraged by having a name with which I could finally move forward. We then tried all the standard medicines and dietary adjustments necessary to treat this condition.

You guessed it – none of them touched my symptoms.

By this point, I was 4 years into my health wilderness. Each year brought at least two ER visits, and the 5th year ended with the Duke doctors giving up. I'll never forget the day I went to his office, and the only suggestion he could offer up was tossing me onto an operating room table, blindly cutting me open for exploratory surgery (not even knowing where to start looking or what to look for). He looked me in the eye and said he had no other options, suggesting I try UNC Chapel Hill or another GI doctor, on the longshot that they had encountered a case like mine at some point.

I was completely broken. I had been strong for so long; I had been a 'fighter' for years, but having one of the best doctors in the country essentially give up on me was among the most discouraging events I've encountered. Naturally, no doctor would say that out loud, but the nonverbal communication was loud and clear.

So, I gave up, too.

Another two years passed, and I learned to live with the daily illness that was now my lifestyle. After trying several naturopathic approaches, supplements, diets, candida cleanses, etc. - none of which were effective - I accepted that I would be sick until the day I die. I grew very angry at God, and pieces of my soul became brittle with resentment and pain. This is obviously not the healthy or recommended approach, but I might as well be brutally honest with you.

Luckily, the story doesn't end there.

One day, I met a man who changed my world (Awww!). He brought levels of encouragement that I had no idea existed. He was confident a cure was somewhere out there, and he always brushed off my certainty that the road would forever be a dead end. In fact, his unwavering certainty was almost annoying, since I had comfortably nestled myself into a cozy pit of misery.

Surrendering to his constant optimism, I caved. The only other option I could brainstorm was a medical facility praised as the best in the country for my condition - the Mayo Clinic. Unfortunately, after spending ungodly amounts with Wake and Duke over the years, I was certain there was no way I would be able to afford such a prestigious name or the travel/lodging that would be required to visit from North Carolina.

In stepped my ever-supportive parents. They had walked with me throughout the entire process and years of doctors, and now, sacrificially offered to fund my last ditch effort. I spent time researching my insurance, finding that Mayo was miraculously covered. We booked the trip, and I flew to Florida.

I entered the facility, bewildered by the massive campus. I snapped a quick photo to share the adventure with my family, but was later tracked down and reprimanded by a security guard for doing so. Oops. Moral of the story: don't take photos inside Mayo. I digress.

Three days in this facility were consumed with constant tests and office visits, all inconclusive. At least many of these tests and possible diagnoses had never before been considered, which was encouraging in itself. They sent me home with a list of tests to complete, hoping something would reveal an answer. No such luck. They then suggested I scale back hours at my horribly stressful job in order to give my body a break.

And what happened when I brought this news back to my supervisors? They fired me. Their disregard for the health situation I was enduring was unbelievable. They informed me that I "may keep my job at part time hours until they hire my replacement, which I'll be expected to train." Well, if that didn't add to the pile in life, I don't know what would. To be fair, I did remain in that position several months longer at part time hours until I left for maternity complications; but that's another story!

I then took up sewing as therapy and something to keep my mind off the struggles I was facing. Soon, I found great passion in making a variety of new products that my friends were begging to own for themselves. Thus, my business was born out of the adversity I endured. I named it Valentia Ifuerza, a derivative of the Spanish translation for "courage and strength."

From aromatherapy spa products, to designer handbags, couture veils, jewelry, baby gifts, and gluten free goodies, my business grew into a successful alternative to the job that had been unceremoniously removed from my grasp. I decided to use my struggles to generate good for others; as business grew, I began donating a portion of the profits to celiac disease research. Please feel free to visit: vi-style.com.

I made my story public, speaking out to local news stations and papers, hoping to shed light on the struggles endured by those with celiac disease. I didn't want all those years of struggle to lead to a dead end anymore, so I am writing this book to give all that pain some purpose. My hope is that this will inspire and help others where it couldn't help me.

Despite a seemingly finished tale, the story's ending brightens.

Shortly after this whole ordeal, my husband and I found out we were expecting twins. This might not seem too remarkable, except that I had been told for years that my illness would keep me from ever conceiving - let alone twins!

As luck would have it, pregnancy did the trick (well, for a bit). After 8 years of every treatment in the book, pregnancy was the only success at curbing my symptoms. About 90% of them cleared up (though replaced by other pregnancy symptoms – which we all know are an entirely different type of fun, but much more tolerable). Even when the relief was only temporary, lasting until birth, I savored every moment.

So as a proud mom and lucky wife, I'd say this story is a

rich success…health or no health.

My plea to you is to take in all the tips and benefit from my experience!

UPDATE: September 2015

My local GI doctor has recently tried a new treatment for the microscopic colitis. This steroid (Uceris brand) has made an immense difference, though there are still good and bad days. Keep heart, GI sufferers! Long journeys can sometimes have lovely views here and there. I'm still by your side.

UPDATE: 2017

I am still on the same steroid, but symptoms return in waves – sometimes quite severe. The journey continues!

the basics

Ok, I'm going to provide a no-nonsense and easy-to-understand overview of what gluten is, how you can avoid it, and if you even NEED to avoid it! I am also going to include a cheat sheet for those of you who are just learning the ropes. Hopefully, this will get you moving toward understanding the world of gluten.

For starters, what in the world is gluten, anyway? Gluten is a protein composite found in a variety of grain products and byproducts. The main culprits are wheat, barley, & rye. Now, the tricky part is that there are often ingredients in your everyday foods that contain gluten; if you don't learn to recognize them, you'll get a sneak attack. Unfortunately, the FDA only requires allergen identification of wheat on labels right now, though we have heard rumors that this may change soon. Until it does, learn what to be on the lookout for! There are also a number of products that have improved labeling "gluten free" on their foods, but not every company is this considerate of our condition. So as much as I'd love to tell you that you can live an easy and brain-dead life, you really do have to educate yourself and become an expert on these ingredients (and therefore, educate those around you so the world is more aware of what we're dealing with).

the main culprits

The following list includes primary sources to avoid. As mentioned, there are a variety of other ingredients by differing names that may be derived from these gluten sources. I will try to include as many of these variations as possible! Download printable cheat sheets at: vi-style.com/gluten.html

wheat
barley
rye
malt/malt flavoring, malt extract, malt vinegar, etc.
durum
semolina
spelt
wheatberries
khorasan wheat (kamut ®)
graham
farina
emmer
einkorn wheat
farro
triticale
triticum

brewer's yeast
wheat starch
bran
chilton
bulgar
thickening agents/roux
crisped rice (like in some candy bars)
fu
heeng
hing
groats
germ
hydrolyzed wheat protein
hordeum vulgare extract
matzo/matza
maida
seitan
perungayam
tabbouleh
tabouli
udon
vital wheat gluten (uh, obviously)

foods that typically contain gluten

breads
cookies
crackers
cakes

pastas
communion wafers
sauces/gravies, particularly anything thickened or a roux
beer
soy sauce
teriyaki sauce
breadcrumbs
brownies (bummer!)
meatballs
casseroles
cookie dough ice cream
cookies & cream ice cream
cream of ____ soups (thickeners)
pizza

foods to proceed with caution and read ingredients

seasonings
sauces
dressings
pre-packaged snacks or side dish mixes
soups
candies
artificial colors (check to see if source is specified – generally safe, but not always)
artificial flavorings (check to see if source is specified – generally safe, but not always)
natural flavor (check to see if source is specified – generally safe, but not always)

coloring (caramel coloring used to be suspicious, but these days it is usually made from corn)
starch, modified food starch (if made in the US, tends to be safe)

celiac disease symptoms

Celiac disease usually presents itself with gastrointestinal upset, though a variety of other symptoms can appear, as well. Each person reacts differently, and there are others who have no signs at all. The most common symptoms include:

diarrhea
bloating
gas
nausea
constipation
cramping
abdominal pain
weight loss
fatigue
skin rash (dermatitis herpetiformis – DH)
nutrient deficiencies
anemia
easy bruising
vertigo
revelation of other autoimmune disorders (thyroid disorders, lactose intolerance, arthritis, etc.)
osteoporosis

dental problems
depression
irritability
joint pain
neuropathy (numbness & tingling)

...and more. If you suffer from any of these symptoms, it might not be a bad idea to have your doctor do a simple blood test for antibodies that may be indicative of celiac disease.

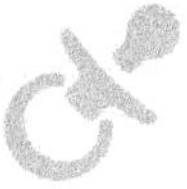

pregnancy, parenting, and gluten

Ah, the life of a mom. From morning sickness, diaper blowouts, and inopportune spit-up attacks…to screaming toddlers, crayons on the wall, and a dog who has recently been painted purple…you have plenty on your plate. Then, someone dares to tell you that this plate can't contain gluten?!

Well, I might not be able to help much with washing Fido or your walls, but health stressors might be something for which a gluten change will do wonders. While converting to a meticulous diet might seem like the last thing you have time for, it might just make your life significantly easier.

A celiac disease diagnosis is confusing enough, but adding the complexity of pregnancy and motherhood will create even more questions than you had before.

Another challenge for the new mother is whether or not to feed her baby gluten as they grow, and if so, when to introduce. This chapter should help answer a lot of your questions.

---

pregnancy & gluten

Bewildered, you pick up that stick just one more time and blink as hard as you can. Pregnancy is overwhelming for anyone, but celiacs get some extra perks. Luckily, I've walked in those shoes – and with TWINS (I'll see your baby and raise you a baby) and a singleton! There are some easy steps to ensure you have a safe experience. Also, take heart. There is some VERY exciting news about pregnancy and celiac disease at the end of this section that could mean monumentally great things for you.

Now, before ever getting pregnant (sorry if I'm too late for some of you), do everything you can to make sure you're being diligent with your gluten free diet. A poorly managed case of celiac disease can lead to fertility issues and might also put the baby at risk for health complications. If you are actively trying to get pregnant, be sure to receive regular testing of your celiac antibodies, as well as all your vital nutrient levels. Sometimes, as you may know, gluten exposure won't show symptoms. This is the most dangerous situation, because you aren't aware anything is wrong, and therefore can't take measures to correct your exposure. When this happens, your vitamin/mineral levels become depleted and at unhealthy levels for you and the baby.

Anyone trying to conceive should already be taking

prenatal vitamins, but it's an especially good idea for anyone with celiac disease. It is also recommended to include an extra folic acid supplement in this regimen, but please contact your doctor for their advice before you proceed with anything I'm suggesting. If you're like me and hate those humongous prenatal pills, I found some great gummy vitamins that encouraged me to keep up the habit. Just be sure that any vitamins you select are gluten free, of course. Companies just love to sneak in little ingredients sometimes, don't they? Hey, it keeps us on our toes.

While having your blood tested, you may also want to request regular monitoring of your iron levels. Anemia is a common complication with celiacs. I had a lot of issues with it prior to pregnancy, and it only worsened once we conceived. Though I took iron supplements, my anemia was so bad that I had to get a two unit blood transfusion when the girls were born. Part of that was also due to an increased amount of blood loss that I experienced with twins.

So, joy! You're having a baby! You inherit…an even stricter diet. Congratulations!

We already know how difficult the gluten free diet is. Now the pregnancy experts tell you to avoid the following:

Undercooked Meats/Eggs/Fish (Yep, Sushi!)

Soft Cheeses (Brie, Feta, etc.)

Unpasteurized Dairy Products

Sandwich Meats

Caffeine (Dangit! Pregnant women could use that more than ANYONE)

Alcohol (Dangit again!)

Fish that are high risk for mercury content

Certain Herbs & Supplements

...and the list goes on. Some of these items are in question by experts, but general suggestion is to avoid them where possible. It's better to be safe than sorry.

I wish I had a quick fix to help with additional dietary restrictions, but I don't. Honestly, the best thing I can say is that it's a bummer – plain and simple - and you aren't alone! I'll be the first to join you for a pity party so we can crack open a bottle of...um...sparkling cider.

I will say this: club soda was a great substitute when I was pregnant (NOT seltzer). I'd never had it before, but mixing it with some orange juice tasted just like a mimosa. When I was craving a beer, it also helped curb that craving. I tried non-alcoholic wine, and did NOT have success. Blech. And do you know how many times my pride was pummeled by anyone I asked about non-alcoholic gluten free beer? They have non-alcoholic beer and they have gluten free beer, but putting the two together is apparently "impossible." We found some obscure versions online, but they were quite difficult to get our hands on. I tried to encourage myself with the knowledge that any such thing would probably taste as bad as licking the inside of my fireplace.

There are plenty of pregnancy books out there with suggestions on how to curb those notorious cravings, especially for junk food. I happen to believe, however, that you should indulge (within reason). Now naturally, you don't want to gain too much weight, causing further health problems down the road. But often times, your body craves things for a reason...plus, what better excuse could one have to indulge than working 24/7 at making a human being from scratch? You earned it, mama! So, considering our celiac lives are defined by what we CAN'T eat, I say find some approved things that make your pregnant belly happy and don't feel guilty one bit if you have a little extra. I had entire meals of bacon my first trimester – ungodly amounts of bacon. Was it the healthiest option? Of course not. But I left the guilt for another time.

Ginger is another godsend. Since we celiacs already have tummy troubles, ginger is a fantastic herbal remedy to ease the discomfort. Add in morning sickness, and it really has its work cut out for it. Local health food stores tend to carry ginger candies that worked wonders for me, in addition to ginger tea. It was helpful for those moments at the office where the nausea hit out of nowhere.

In addition to ginger, peppermint has a similar effect. To this day, I find the best quick aid for a queasy stomach is a strong peppermint gum. There are also many who swear by the use of essential oils, suggesting a variety of ways peppermint oil can also help. Bring up some of these natural solutions to your doctor, making sure it isn't a concern for your baby.

My last tip for dealing with pregnancy nausea is "little eating." Spread out very small meals throughout your day, and add healthy snacks in between. This also helps curb cravings, keeping you from eating too many of the junk foods you shouldn't. If you're like me, I was constantly on the go, so this wasn't always easy to do. Stock your purse, office, car, and bedside table with water and snacks. The more you keep your stomach from ever going completely empty, the better chance you'll have at avoiding morning sickness. Some people even set alarms twice during the night to wake up and have a GF granola bar; they swear it keeps them from having any issues in the morning. I mention keeping water nearby because staying well hydrated will also help with your nausea.

---

labor & delivery

The time comes for your little one to make his big debut.

A few weeks prior to delivery, there are some great steps you can take to avoid tough situations during one of the happiest times of your life. As a celiac, sometimes planning ahead is your best friend. Here are some live-and-learn tips that will make all the difference so you can relax and enjoy the experience.

When packing your hospital bag, include plenty of gluten free snacks and ready-to-eat meal alternatives. Pack enough snacks for dad, too. He is there round-the-clock just like you and will need his own stash!

Make a lot of pre-made gluten free meals for your freezer. That might also include a bag of ingredients you can toss in the Crock Pot for your favorite recipe. Staying well stocked is a great idea, but keep in mind that if you plan to breastfeed, you may want to leave some free space in your freezer to store breast milk.

Also, all those well-meaning friends and family who constantly say "Let us know if you need anything!" will be able to put those words into action. Send out some easy GF recipes they can keep on hand to make once the baby arrives. They might not understand the whole 'gluten' thing, but if you send simple recipes, there's a foolproof way they can help out. Better yet, have them buy this book for a great list of recipe options (plus, they might learn something)!

When touring the hospital in your third trimester, see

> if they'll let you speak with the kitchen supervisor and staff dieticians about what options they make available. Even going to these lengths, I hate to tell you that it may not help much. You end up telling 20 different cafeteria employees about your restrictions, and your tray still has cold pancakes plopped right in the middle.
>
> Be that as it may, my plan-ahead suggestion is to also email friends and family a list of several restaurants close to the hospital and what items from their menu you know are safe to eat. Then, when your biscuits and gravy arrive from the hospital kitchen, you can make a quick call to your best friend to bail you & dad out with some real food.

Now, to the fantastic news I promised you. In all the years of doctors, treatments, medicines, tests, etc., I told you I never received relief. I was still having severe symptoms, even with a strict gluten free diet, and no one could figure out any methods to calm down my symptoms.

Pregnancy did the trick! After 7 years, this season of carrying a baby finally brought my lower GI tract to a place of peace. It didn't happen immediately. In fact, I believe it didn't happen until I was well into my second trimester. I held my breath each day, trying not to jinx the magic. This good health continued until I stopped breastfeeding. Even though it only lasted a season, I'm not sure if I've ever been so thankful for anything in my life. Unfortunately, my second pregnancy didn't follow suit, but each pregnancy is different. I'll take what I can get – thank you, God!

I'm not the only one with this story. I have two other friends with extremely similar health pasts to my own, both of whom had the same success for the same time period. Their stories are featured in our last chapter, so be sure to check it out. Hopefully, if you have had similar problems, you might have a little bit of relief with pregnancy! Now, to figure out how to stay pregnant all the time…

---

breastfeeding & first foods

You've now brought home your beautiful baby – what's next? Science indicates children of a celiac parent(s) are at much higher risk for being genetically predisposed to celiac disease than that of other children. It doesn't mean they're destined for it, though. There are also steps parents can take to make sure a gluten-free life doesn't have to be as hard for our children as it sounds.

One thing doctors agree on is the benefits of breastfeeding, particularly with a baby at risk of celiac disease. There are also theories that the amount of time a baby consumes breast milk can be related to their chances at contracting celiac disease. Breast milk, with its long list of nutritive and beneficial properties, has always been praised as 'the best way to go.' It may not be the best way for you and your baby, though. Sometimes the stars don't align and everyone can't breastfeed - that's okay! I can't produce very much, so that's always been a struggle, but every little bit helps.

It took a lot of work for my flat-chested little self to get the milk flowing, and even so, keeping up with the demand of twin babies became more than I was able to handle. Sure, if I fed them every three hours, and then staggered that with pumping every two hours, I was golden! Not only is that an impossible schedule for anyone that requires sleep to live, but it's also exhausting for people who are already up at all hours with new babies.

But hey, at least at this point, you aren't pregnant anymore, so you can have all the coffee you want to help the situation! Oh…no…wait. Not while you're breastfeeding. How cruel.

I was fortunate enough to have a close friend who was also an extremely knowledgeable lactation expert, Jamilla Walker, of the Labor Ladies (thelaborladies.com). She offered me some fantastic tips, as well as recipes for lactation cookies that helped with my milk supply. Be sure to see one of these recipes, included in our dessert section!

I made it as long as I could, and finally gave up. Luckily, some very close friends of ours were selfless enough to become milk donors for our family. It sounds awkward and perhaps a little gross - accepting milk from your friend's boob - but it ended up not being strange at all, and such an unspeakable blessing. If you DO end up being someone who found GI relief during pregnancy and breastfeeding, I strongly urge you to become a milk donor to keep your relief going as long as possible. There are also a lot of moms in need who would treasure the chance at some nutrient-rich breast milk for their babies.

introducing food

There are various studies claiming you can prevent celiac disease by introducing gluten to a child's diet at just the right time. Some doctors and scholars say there is a magic window between 5 and 7 months that will help prevent the onset of the disease. Others say to introduce it as early as possible. And even others still, claim to wait as long as possible to introduce it, delaying its onset. At this point, none of these positions has enough evidence to support its claim. Generally accepted opinion tends to lean toward gradually introducing gluten in that 5 to 7 month window. I did this with my babies, but we don't know enough in the medical world yet to confirm if this was the right choice. I'll let you know if they become celiac!

---

gf parenting

As your child grows, watch for the typical symptoms that are often misdiagnosed. Among many, the main ones that present in young children are:

Diarrhea

Vomiting

Failure to Gain Weight

Distended (Swollen) Belly

Slowed Growth

Lethargy

Be sure to stay up-to-date on pediatrician visits and make sure they're on the lookout for celiac disease symptoms, as well.

Once your child does receive a positive diagnosis, all is not lost! It's true that controlling the diet of a child can be more difficult than that of an adult, but there are ways to make the experience easier. Be thankful you were diligent and caught the illness early, as this eliminates a lot of dangerous complications that could've happened.

While your child is still young, controlling the foods he encounters is much easier. Watch your ingredient labels carefully, as many baby foods and toddler snacks sneak wheat and other gluten into the products.

As your child grows, begin training them about what is safe and what isn't – it's never too early. As soon as they begin talking, it is already a good time to get them understanding. It's also going to be crucial for the day they leave your house for preschool or to stay with a friend/babysitter. While your child certainly won't be responsible enough to be able to do much about it, sometimes quizzing them in "ok foods" and "not ok foods" can make a huge difference to avoid an accidental ingestion by a teacher or caregiver.

One thing I suggest is creating a mantra. Kids memorize things easily with those fresh little brains, and repetition is the best way to ingrain important things. Maybe even make a rhyme.

> My name is Sarah, and I can run quick!
>
> I can't eat gluten 'cause I'll get really sick.
>
> Gluten is in wheat, barley, sometimes oats, and rye.
>
> Keep those things away so we stay healthy, you and I!

I'm sure you can think up something infinitely better than that, but you get the idea. As they get older, turn it into a game. Hold up flash cards with a picture of food (cupcakes, brownies, bananas, etc.) – both safe foods and unsafe foods – and have the kids learn which are safe and which aren't. This little bit of independence helps as they are in more activities and schooling away from home, where you can't watch them 24/7.

Which brings me to my next tip. Have an easy-to-read form letter ready to go anytime your child has a new teacher, coach, etc. so they can help your child avoid dangerous situations. This letter should be very friendly (you ARE asking them for help, after all – help that falls outside their realm of expertise and comfort), but also indicative of the severity this health issue poses. Many view the avoidance of gluten as a fad diet or a hippie parent choice, and have no idea that it can put a child's life at risk. Take a look at the form letter / cheat sheet I have created for these circumstances. I have made it available for download so you may edit it to suit your situation. It all fits on one page so it's a simple reference they may keep handy throughout the year. Print out your single-sheet version at vi-style.com/gluten.html.

Gluten Cheat Sheet for Teachers, Coaches, Etc.

First and foremost, thank you so much for all you do for our child!

We know how full your plate already is, so we apologize for heaping on one more thing. We greatly appreciate your help in keeping our child from extreme illness or even a hospital trip. You may be familiar with how peanut or dairy allergies work, but our child's celiac disease (response to gluten) can be just as life-threatening. Contrary to popular belief, it isn't a fad diet; it's an actual diagnosis that makes him very sick when he comes in contact with even the smallest crumb of something that was made with wheat, barley, rye, and anything derived from these grains. That also means if someone laid bread on his plate and quickly remembered the allergy...he still needs a new plate. Please know this isn't us trying to be a pain in the neck - it's how this extremely sensitive allergy actually works. Trust me, we hate it, too!

Here is a VERY shortened and basic list containing examples of safe and unsafe foods/snacks. The real list is quite long, so we are trying to make this a little easier to reference. Be on the watch for some of these type foods:

UNSAFE
Crackers
Bread
Flour (crafting/cooking)
Cookies
Pizza
Pasta
Cake
Most Cereals
Brownies
Soy Sauce
Many marinades/spices/dressings
Gravy or thickened sauces (flour)

GENERALLY SAFE
Salt & Pepper as seasoning
Clean meats (no added

marinades/sauces/spices/gravy)
Clean vegetables (no added marinades/sauces/spices/gravy)
Fruit
Rice
Potatoes
Fruit snacks
Foods labeled as "gluten free" on packaging
Sweets and candies that don't contain wheat/barley/rye in ingredients (check label on all of these - they can be tricky)
Salads (no croutons or pita chips added)

When parents bring off-limits treats to class, we hope you may use the treat stash we have given you so that our child can have something tasty to enjoy, too.

You can imagine how scary it is to release our child into the world when he has to battle such a tough allergy. It's also very hard for our child to watch others eat "normal" food and feel left out (especially when fitting in at school can be tough for everyone). We certainly don't want to make waves in your everyday activities, but anywhere you can accommodate our child and help him be able to be included is SO appreciated. Hopefully this cheat sheet is something you can keep on hand as a reference for helping our child.

Again, thank you for all you do in our child's life and for helping us keep him healthy!

This letter is also great to email another parent before your kid embarks on a sleepover or birthday party. You'll notice I mention the scenario of parents bringing treats to class. A worthwhile solution can be to send some sort of non-perishable gluten free treat (maybe packaged cookies or your child's favorite candy?) that your child can enjoy while the other students have theirs. I recognize it isn't the same, but at least it can help soften the child from feeling too left out. Perhaps you can also create little cards for teachers to use that say "We enjoyed ____ treat today. Unfortunately, it wasn't safe for Sarah, but I can vouch that she earned an equally exciting treat for later!" Leave a line for the teacher to sign, and allow your child a special treat once they get home. These are just a couple ideas, but find something that works for your child and go for it!

The last daunting area when raising a gf child is the lunchroom. Most often, cafeteria staff are not properly trained in what gluten is or how to provide a clean meal for your child. Here are some tips on keeping your child's lunchtime safe:

> The obvious solution would be to pack all their lunches. This is not only a pain for you, but it can make the child feel left out – never getting to buy his lunch.
>
> Work with administrators to see if you can create an approved list of meals that can be put together from what is already in their pantry.
>
> Offer to give an easy 1-hour class to their kitchen staff on the basics of gluten – what it is, what foods contain it, and what can happen to your child if they

ingest it.

Print out and laminate the cheat sheets from "the basics" chapter of this book, so they may post it as a reference in their kitchen.

Visit the cafeteria periodically with your child (if parents still do that these days) and order a gluten free meal to see what game plan is in place. Ask staff if they are able to identify your child and automatically make sure his food is gluten free without him having to ask every day.

Some schools are willing to be quite accommodating, but there are other schools that are more resistant to anything that makes their job a little more difficult. In the event you encounter some administrators who aren't willing to make these reasonable accommodations, there are ways to be more firm with your message.

I'm no lawyer, but I've done my fair share of reading on the topic. Celiac disease is considered a disability, and therefore, a protected class in situations like this. There is a Federal law in place requiring schools to make dietary accommodations for students with celiac disease. Hopefully, all it will take is explaining this fact to administrators (along with a signed doctor's note confirming the diagnosis and dietary requirements) to get your point across. If you still encounter resistance, it might not be a bad idea to involve an attorney for advice on your child's rights. It is my understanding, however, that gluten *sensitivity* (vs. celiac disease) may not be covered by these laws.

As your children grow, becoming more independent, they will be able to watch their own diet. Teenagers tend to succumb to the pressures of wanting to fit in. Even when they are aware of what foods to avoid, sometimes social situations make them uncomfortable with food complications. Many parents see a symptom recurrence in the teenage years when eating like a 'normal person' avoids them a tough social situation. Sometimes, as they re-introduce gluten, they don't even have symptoms for a while. This can be most dangerous, because they see no reason to be gluten free when they feel just fine eating it. Be sure to constantly check in with your teen, reminding them how important the diet is to their current and long-term health.

the ‘hit’ list

You’re embarking on your first visit to the healthy grocery store, and you find yourself dizzy with various options and sky high prices. Not knowing where to start, you wander into the baking aisle, only to find 15 different brands of gluten free all-purpose baking flours. Which one will have a similar consistency to what you’re used to? Which will rise properly? Which will cook evenly? Which will taste like ground toenails (most of them)? And then you ask yourself, “Do I even need to be shopping here or can I get this stuff at my usual store?”

It’s a daunting task, but we did all the dirty work for you. We taste tested for years and wasted money on products we should’ve left on the shelf. We believe our pain shouldn’t be in vain, so I’ve teamed up with fellow celiacs to provide you our list of favorite GF packaged products for various purposes. Though everyone has personal preferences (and you’ll still have some trial and error on your own to see what fits your tastes), we hope to at least get you off to the right start.

substitution basics

Though the healthy supermarkets are a great place to get some specialty items, your staple foods should still come from your favorite store. In your transition to GF life, your main diet should consist of cleanly cooked meats & vegetables, minimizing your starches to items like potatoes or rice. You'll find yourself feeling a lot better the less starches you pack in, and you typically adopt a healthier body when you eat this way. There are a variety of diets out there that build upon this concept (Paleo, Atkins, etc.), but the extremes aren't always necessary in order to fuel a healthy lifestyle.

One of the biggest mistakes people make when they go gluten free is simply walking into a health food store and buying up every gluten free item they find, therefore gaining a tremendous amount of weight. Why do they gain? Well, think about it. Most stores don't label meats, vegetables, and fresh foods as gluten free, because it's pretty obvious that they are. It's the baked goods and replacement foods that get gluten replacements - cakes, cookies, crackers, pastas, breads, etc. If you fill your diet with all THOSE foods, you're destined for a weight/health disaster! Even non-GF people would be in serious trouble if they only ate baked goods, pastas, and breads for every meal.

As if that weren't enough, you'll notice that a lot of gluten free replacement foods are much higher in fat and calories than their glutinous counterparts. Why? As mentioned, many GF substitute grains taste like ground toenails or dirty feet. In order to mask this problem, companies pile on the sugar, butter, and flavorings so you don't notice what you're missing by eating gluten free. These cover-ups cause a spike in calories and fats, thereby increasing your waistline and health risks.

So, definitely be wary of this as you decide how much of your diet will receive GF substitutes. This problem can also present itself with those who are uneducated to the reasons for a gluten free diet, thereby adopting it as a fad diet (thinking it will make them lose weight). While these people might make some of us furious ("Hey, if you CAN eat the foods, why in the world wouldn't you?! No one WANTS to live this way!"), they can also provide a benefit to us. The more demand that exists for gluten free foods (even from these people), the more companies will meet that demand with further options we can choose from and more carefully developed, better tasting/performing products.

I should also note that there are some who adopt the diet in the appropriate way, which can encourage a healthier lifestyle. I won't get into the debate here, but there is research to support a belief that today's grains are so genetically altered, they are no longer recognizable to the human body, therefore being treated as an alien substance to attack. These researchers believe many of our world's auto-immune diseases are caused and/or affected by these foods. I won't take a side here, but it's an interesting topic to read up on…you know, in all your spare time!

---

where to go

A surprisingly great place to find GF packaged foods is actually Walmart. They have a wide selection of pastas and baking supplies. Sometimes they have a separate gluten free section, and in other store locations, the items are sprinkled in among the shelves. Either way, the prices are much more reasonable than a specialty store. And hey, you can pick up a garden hose and craft supplies in the same trip!

When I refer to products found at my local grocery store, that would be Harris Teeter. I believe this chain is only in certain states along the east coast, but perhaps you have a similar grocer near you. I feel HT is getting much better with carrying gluten free options, but your stores may be different. Food Lion and Aldi are other chains that have increased their GF supplies, while also being known for affordable prices.

It should be noted that I haven't received any sort of compensation for featuring anything here by brand or location. These are simply my unfiltered suggestions for you! Keep in mind that you have to get a feel to what baking techniques/temperatures/times work best for your situation. Often times when baking gluten-free foods, you'll find the frustrating issue that your pan of brownies or cake have burned around the edges, but are still gooey/liquid in the middle. Sometimes you have to make your own adjustments, but keep a watch for this as you bake gluten free.

Some favorite products:

General baking mix: Pamela's Baking & Pancake Mix (I make pancakes at least once a week with this and love it. It also makes a nice substitute for flour in many recipes. It has the best flavor of anything I've found). This is my #1 must-have and I simply cannot live without it. I'd say it is worth the price more than any other GF product on the market. Good work, Pam.

All-purpose flour: Pamela's "Cup for Cup" Flour

Crackers: Glutino "table crackers."

Snack Crackers: Van's "Say Cheese" and Multi-grain Crackers, found at WalMart. We also enjoy Nabisco's White Cheddar GF Rice Thins. A lot of rice crackers have a funny burnt taste, so watch out for that. Lance has also recently released a GF "Ritz Bitz" style sandwich cracker. 5 stars, people!

Bread (for toasting or drying into breadcrumbs): Udi's White Bread – found in our local grocery store, and at health food stores

Bread (untoasted for sandwiches and the like): Canyon Bakehouse brand, found at Target. I prefer the multi-grain to the white, but to each his own.

Bagels: Promise brand Cinnamon Raisin Bagels

Homemade Bread Mix: Pamela's Bread Mix

Pasta brands: Schar (Bonta d' Italia) and Walmart brand (Great Value). Most pastas are gritty, mushy, stuck together, poor taste, etc.; you name it. We always include some oil in our pasta water to help with the sticking issue; then, throughout cooking, I like to keep pulling pieces apart by using a fork to stir. Most GF brands suggest you rinse well with cold water after cooking. I find that this helps even for the brands that don't say to do so. It pulls the leftover starch off the noodles so they aren't as mushy. Yes, it's a pain to have cold pasta, but adding your hot pasta sauce immediately or a quick pop in the microwave will get you back in business.

Cake Mix: I was a fan of Gluten Free Pantry's spice cake mix, but it seems to have disappeared from local store shelves. Pamela's also makes a decent cake mix. Betty Crocker is good for certain recipes and tends to be more readily available at the local store. Just be aware: most GF cake mixes only end up making half the cake that a normal mix produces. Namaste is one brand that gives you a full mix amount (two 9" round pans), but it does cost a bit more.

Cookie Mix: Betty Crocker. Their chocolate chip cookies and sugar cookies are pretty fabulous and readily available at many grocery stores. I add some extra sugar to the sugar cookie mix, and cinnamon for amazing snickerdoodles. To die for!

Ready-Made Cookies: Glutino and Pamela's do a pretty good job with this, though some of the cookie types are better than others within these two brands. MI-DEL also makes great ginger snaps and chocolate chip cookies, while being easy to find and keeping a reasonable price point. Whole Foods Gluten Free Bakehouse in the frozen foods aisle has some delicious choices, too.

Brownie Mix: Betty Crocker. I always added mini chocolate chips to my brownies until these came along. Now they include those for me! Be careful – there are many GF brownie brands that are chalky and…well…gross. Most brands also make half the amount of standard brownie mixes.

Cornbread Mix: Bob's Red Mill

Toaster Pastries: Glutino. And they finally added frosting! Hooray!

Cereals: The gluten-free Chex options (rice, in particular), are always a winning choice. I also applaud Cheerios for joining the GF team for many of their cereals! Gorilla Munch by EnviroKids is also a good choice for kids.

Hot Cereals: Growing up, I used to eat Cream of Wheat for breakfast any mornings we were sick. They have recently developed Cream of Rice, and it's a wonderful substitute. And if you're southern, grits are always the way to go (just avoid cross-contamination).

Breadcrumbs: I haven't found an incredibly successful mass-produced breadcrumb. Being a southerner, our recipes and casseroles seem to all have breadcrumbs, so I typically either dry out some Udi's and throw it in the food processor, or I grind Glutino "table crackers" (not the round ones). It works flawlessly for me!

Beer: Redbridge, by Anheuser Busch, tends to be a crowd favorite. I also enjoy bottled hard ciders when around other friends with beer. Some of them are extremely sweet (Woodchuck, Angry Orchard), yet I'm a fan of a drier cider (Crispin

Original Flavor and Original Sin). Crispin also has a honey crisp flavor, which is very dark/thick cider, mimicking a stout beer. My personal favorite cider these days is Johnny Appleseed. It's well balanced.

Liquor: For years, I only drank potato vodkas since most liquors are derived from glutinous grains. But researches claimed along the way that the distilling process actually disables the protein in gluten, rendering it harmless to celiacs. You may like to do your own research on the topic, but it's generally accepted that many liquors are safe to drink. But be warned: alcohol in general can worsen your GI symptoms.

Ready-Made Pie Crusts: Whole Foods brand Gluten Free Bakehouse in the frozen section. It comes with two crusts, which cook up wonderfully and taste fantastic. My (non-gf) mother even uses these over her traditional crusts because of their great flavor.

Ready-Made Biscuits: Whole Foods brand Gluten Free Bakehouse in the frozen section. They have regular cream biscuits and cheddar biscuits.

Ready-Made Banana Bread and Carrot Cake: Whole Foods brand Gluten Free Bakehouse in the frozen section.

Hamburger and Hot Dog Buns: I'm starting to think this search is a lost cause. I have tried nearly every brand that exists, and though some aren't as bad as others (you will find lots of hockey pucks), none have been worth my time. I end up just being happier eating mine naked. Some friends even put them on gf sandwich bread. I say "to each his own" on this one, and Godspeed.

Donuts: Kinnikinnick frozen donuts. They're a little expensive, considering you only get a few in a pack, but the cinnamon-sugar ones have been a delicious substitute for us.

Baby Snacks: Happypuffs brand. We also use most any brand of the yogurt melts and freeze dried veggie snacks. Just check the ingredients well, naturally.

Granola Bars: I enjoy KIND bars (if you prefer a chunkier trail mix style) and Larabars (for the soft/fruity style). There are many GF granola options available, but I have tried some nasty ones in my days. I don't eat them often, but I do know that they're getting better across the board.

Cream of Mushroom Soup: I use this in many recipes. Pacific Foods makes a great GF cream of mushroom, and Progresso has now made their cream of mushroom gluten free. As far as availability and affordability, both work great.

Soy Sauce: San-J makes a wonderful GF soy sauce – aka tamari sauce – that is also available as low-sodium, organic, and to-go packets.

Naturally, you may do your own taste-tests to see what works best for your family. New products are arriving daily, so I'm excited to keep trying and exploring. This list may become out of date as the gluten free world evolves, so I will try my best to update much of this on our website: vi-style.com.

gf chef

Show of hands, who has picked up a gluten free cookbook and gotten nauseous at the thought of how much they will spend on ingredients for one homemade bread recipe? How about trying to collect obscure ingredients to help your dish mimic the real world ("Xanthan gum? What is that?")? What about those of you who have tried to alter your favorite recipe, only to find that GF flours don't respond like normal flour and you end up with some sort of disastrous oven volcano or half-baked shoe-tasting mess?

I've been there. So, I collected some of my favorite recipes that are extremely simple and relatively inexpensive. In fact, almost all of these contain ingredients I can pick up at my local grocery store. As we mentioned before, the name of the game is cooking with meats and vegetables wherever possible, dodging GF substitutes unless necessary. This is a peek inside my family's most prized recipes, none of which will disappoint (thanks to my talented mom and grandmas)! Feel like the holidays have lost that special something? I've included our Thanksgiving and Christmas favorites, all adapted into a delectable GF version. You won't know the difference! Some of my closest gluten free friends have also contributed recipes that you won't want to miss.

Recipes include:

Appetizers:
Sausage Balls
Buffalo Chicken Dip
Mini Frittatas
Pineapple Lemon Cream

Main Dishes:
Parmesan Chicken
Pasta Primavera
Chicken Noodle Casserole
Seasoned Chicken
Chicken Stew
Vegetable Beef Stew
Chicken Casserole
Chilly Day Chili
Swiss Chicken
Sirloin Tips
Irresistible Spaghetti
Beef Stroganoff
Shrimp Fried Rice
Mexican Lasagna

Side Dishes:
Parmesan Seasoned New Potatoes
Squash Casserole
Thanksgiving Stuffing/Dressing
Sweet Potato Soufflé
Mixed Vegetable Casserole
Cheesy Grits Soufflé
Cheesy Baked Macaroni
Broccoli Casserole
Pineapple Casserole
Cranberry Jello Salad
Lime Jello Salad
Carrot Salad
Mexican Rice & Beans

Desserts:
Angel Food Cake
Strawberry Cobbler
Pumpkin Pie
Peppermint Snowball Truffles
Oatmeal Raisin Cookies
Milkin' Cookies (Lactation)
No Bake Cookies
Gooey Cake
Million Dollar Pie
Simple Cheesecake
Chocolate Cherry Cookies

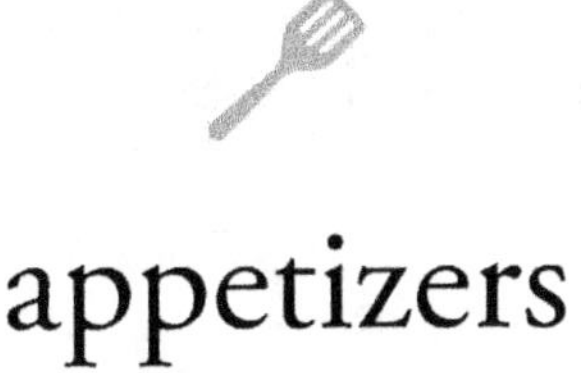

appetizers

sausage balls

1 lb. regular sausage
12 oz. sharp cheddar grated cheese
2 tbsp. dried basil
3 c. Pamela's Baking Mix

Mix all ingredients well. I use a food processor, but your hands will work just fine, too (it takes a lot longer). Roll dough into balls – roughly 1 to 1.5 inch – and place on cookie sheet (with lip, so that grease doesn't leak into oven).

Bake at 350 degrees for 15 minutes

Recipe Contributor: Rosemary Watts
GF Adaptation: Lauren Hatfield

buffalo chicken dip

2/3 c. buffalo sauce
3/4 c. blue cheese dressing
2 blocks of cream cheese, well softened
24oz shredded chicken
1 c. grated sharp cheddar cheese

Mix all ingredients well & place in a 9"x13" baking dish.

Bake at 350 degrees for 20-25 minutes

Recipe Contributor: Lauren Hatfield

mini frittatas

12-15 eggs (will depend on your cups)
seasoning to taste (seasoned salt, garlic salt, onion salt, italian seasoning, pepper, etc.)
1-2 c. grated cheddar cheese
3 green onions, finely diced
chopped bacon

We highly recommend using silicone baking cups. If you use paper cups, prepare for sticking. If using metal tins, spray well with nonstick spray.

Whisk eggs well with seasoning. Sprinkle a small amount of bacon in the bottom of your baking cups, followed by a sprinkle of cheddar cheese and green onions. Pour egg mixture (preferably from a spout/pitcher) over each baking cup until 3/4 full. Use a fork to lightly stir each cup.

Bake at 375 degrees for 25-35 minutes until just starting to turn golden.

*Great to cook ahead of time and refrigerate. Pull out and heat for a quick on-the-go breakfast or snack. You may substitute the bacon, green onions, and cheese, depending on your taste.

Recipe Contributor: Lauren Hatfield

pineapple lemon cream

1 small can crushed pineapple, with juice
1/2 c. sugar
1 block of cream cheese, well softened
1 small box of lemon jell-o
1 8oz. tub of whipped cream

Bring pineapple (with juice) and sugar to a boil. Add jell-o packet and stir well. Remove from heat. Add cream cheese and combine well with a mixer. Add whipped cream, and combine again with your mixer. Pour into serving dish and refrigerate at least 4 hours until set.

Recipe Contributor: Rosemary Watts

main dishes

parmesan chicken

2-4 deboned chicken breasts
1 stick (1/2 c.) melted butter
Glutino table crackers (not round crackers) – 1/2 box
1/2 c. grated parmesan cheese

Finely grind crackers in food processor with grated cheese (you may sub GF breadcrumbs or dry out some Udi's bread to grind into crumbs). Dip each piece of chicken in the melted butter, then roll in breadcrumb/cheese mixture until well coated. Lay in a baking dish. After all chicken breasts have been coated, feel free to sprinkle a bit of the leftover crumb mixture and butter over entire baking dish.

Bake at 350 degrees for 30-45 minutes or until chicken is cooked through.

Serve either as a main dish with vegetables, or serve next to your favorite gf pasta and red sauce for a heavenly Italian Chicken Parmesan.

Recipe Contributor: Rosemary Watts
GF Adaptation: Lauren Hatfield

pasta primavera

1 small onion, finely diced
4-5 garlic cloves, minced
1/4 c. olive oil (roughly)
3 tbsp. butter
1 bag of baby spinach
1 container grape tomatoes, half sliced
1 container of fresh mushrooms, sliced
1 package of gf spaghetti or gf angel hair pasta
1 tbsp fresh dried/ground basil or italian seasoning
salt & pepper to taste

Sautee all ingredients but spinach for about 20 minutes, until well reduced. Cook pasta according to package instructions. Add spinach to sauce about 5 minutes prior to serving, stirring in well. Combine sauce with noodles and serve with grated parmesan cheese.

Recipe Contributor: Lauren Hatfield

chicken noodle casserole

2-3 chicken breasts: cooked & shredded
1package of Schar brand tagliatelle pasta (broken gf fettuccini noodles will work, as well)
1/2 c. chopped celery
1/3 c. chopped green pepper
1/3 c. chopped onion
1/2 tsp. salt
1 tbsp. chopped pimiento
1 c. mayonnaise
1 can cream of mushroom soup (not concentrated)
1 c. shredded cheddar cheese
1/2 c. milk (if needed)

Cook noodles according to package instructions. Combine all ingredients and stir well. If your soup is extra thick and the mixture seems to need a little extra milk to thin, add up to 1/2 c.

Bake at 350 degrees for 30 minutes or until bubbly.

Recipe Contributor: Rosemary Watts
GF Adaptation: Lauren Hatfield

seasoned chicken

chicken breasts
italian seasoning
onion salt
garlic powder
seasoning salt
1/2 Goya seasoning packet (con azafran/saffron)
salt
pepper

This recipe is not only extremely easy, quick, and delicious, but it's also quite flexible. You'll notice I didn't put any measurements next to my ingredients, because you may alter this recipe to your family's size/taste. Lightly dust each seasoning on the chicken – both sides. Place in a baking dish and bake until chicken has cooked through. I always recommend foil on top with corners slightly depressed inward to keep the chicken juicy.

Bake at 350 degrees for 30-45 minutes, or until cooked throughout.

Recipe Contributor: Lauren Hatfield

chicken stew

4 chicken breasts, containing bone & skin
2 stalks celery
1 onion, halved
3 tbsp. Pamela's cup for cup flour (or any gf flour)
3/4-1c. cold water
1 large can of evaporated milk
milk
2 tbsp. butter

Cook chicken with celery and onion for approximately 30 minutes. Remove chicken from pot; debone & shred. Remove celery & onion from broth. Mix the flour with 3/4c. – 1c. cold water until smooth. Add to hot broth, stirring constantly. Bring to low boil for 1-2 minutes, still stirring constantly. Add evaporated milk and shredded chicken to pot. Add butter and fill the rest of the pot with regular milk (leave a little room to avoid spilling over).

Low simmer at least 1 hour, stirring often to avoid burned milk and boil-over.

Recipe Contributor: Alice Settle
GF Adaptations: Lauren Hatfield

vegetable beef stew

1 lb. stew beef
1 onion, finely chopped
1 large can of petite diced tomatoes, with juice
3 c. water
2 tbsp. tomato paste
1 small bag frozen mixed vegetables
1 small bag of fresh baby potatoes
salt & pepper to taste

Cut stew beef into bite sized pieces, and brown in pot with onions and a splash of vegetable oil (to avoid sticking/burning). Add tomatoes, water, tomato paste, and salt/pepper; return to full boil. Add mixed vegetables and return to a boil while stirring. Allow to simmer on low heat at least 1 hour, but often is more flavorful the longer you can simmer. Quarter baby potatoes and add to soup about a half hour prior to serving. Taste to reassess your salt/pepper needs.

Recipe Contributor: Rosemary Watts

classic chicken casserole

2 boiled chicken breasts, shredded or finely chopped
8 oz. frozen mixed vegetables, cooked
2 c. shredded cheddar cheese (1 bag)
1 small onion, finely chopped
3/4 c. mayonnaise
1/2 c. non-concentrated GF cream of mushroom soup
1 tsp. salt (or to taste)
2 tbsp. melted butter
buttered GF breadcrumbs (or well crushed GF crackers)

Combine first 7 ingredients and pour into 9"x13" baking dish. Top with buttered GF breadcrumbs.

Bake at 350 degrees for 30 minutes

Recipe Contributor: Lauren Hatfield

chilly day chili

2 lb. ground beef
2 onions, finely chopped
1 tsp. oregano
1 tbsp. chili powder
1 tbsp cumin
2 28 oz. cans petite diced tomatoes, with juice
1 can of kidney beans, drained
1 1/2 c. red wine
1 small can tomato paste
splash of hot sauce...or lots of it. your funeral.
1 tsp. garlic powder
1/2 tsp. onion powder
salt & pepper to taste

Brown ground beef and onions in a pot; then drain, if necessary. Add other ingredients and return to boil for 1 minute, stirring well. Add water if chili seems too thick. Simmer on low heat for an hour to 5 hours.

Recipe Contributor: Lauren Hatfield

swiss chicken

chicken breasts, boneless & skinless
slices of swiss cheese (also works well with mozzarella)
3/4 can non-concentrated GF cream of mushroom soup
1/4 c. white wine
1 cup GF breadcrumbs
2 tbsp. italian seasoning
2-3 tbsp. melted butter (optional)

For GF breadcrumbs, I recommend drying out Udi's GF white bread and chopping in the food processor. Add Italian seasoning to your breadcrumbs and mix well. Place chicken in baking dish, adding a generous layer of sliced cheese on top. Stir together soup & wine, then pour or spoon over dish. Sprinkle seasoned breadcrumbs on top, then drizzle with melted butter (optional). I always recommend foil on top with corners slightly depressed inward to keep the chicken juicy. This dish pairs nicely with rice or mashed potatoes, using leftover sauce as a delectable gravy.

Bake at 350 degrees for 30-45 minutes or until chicken has cooked through.

Recipe Contributor: Rosemary Watts
GF Adaptations: Lauren Hatfield

sirloin tips

2 tbsp. butter
2 lbs. beef sirloin tips, cut into bite size cubes
1 can GF beef stock
1/3 c. red wine
1 tbsp. GF soy sauce (San-J makes a great one)
dash of garlic powder
1/4 tsp. onion salt
2 tbsp. corn starch (optional)
1/4 c. water

Mix corn starch and beef stock well and set aside. Melt butter in large skillet. Brown meat, then add broth mixture and other ingredients

Simmer on low heat for 30 minutes, or until meat is tender.

Recipe Contributor: Lauren Hatfield

irresistible spaghetti

1 lb. ground chuck
medium onion, finely chopped
green pepper, finely chopped
garlic, if desired
6 oz. can tomato paste (mixed with 3 c. hot water)
1/2 tsp. oregano
1 tsp. salt (more or less to taste)
1/4 tsp. pepper (more or less to taste)
1 tsp. italian seasoning
1 small can petite diced tomatoes, with juice
1 package GF spaghetti pasta (Schar "Bonta d' Italia" is great)

Brown ground beef with onion and green pepper. Pour off excess grease. Add other ingredients and simmer at least 1 hour (the longer the better). Cook noodles according to package instructions, and combine with sauce.

Recipe Contributor: Alice Settle
GF Adaptations: Lauren Hatfield

beef stroganoff

1-1 1/2 lbs. stew beef (or ground beef)
1 package GF tagliatelle pasta by Schar or broken GF fettuccini pasta
2 tbsp. oil
1 can non-condensed GF cream of mushroom soup
6 oz. sour cream
1 package of fresh mushrooms, sliced

Prepare pasta as directed on package. Fry beef and mushrooms in a skillet with oil. Combine drained pasta with beef, soup, and sour cream. Season to taste. Best served the next day.

Recipe Contributor: Lauren Hatfield

shrimp fried rice

1 lb boiled shrimp, deboned, shelled, tails removed
3c cooked white rice (we use jasmine rice, but sushi rice or your favorite will do fine)
2 eggs
1c frozen peas & carrots, cooked
1 tsp fresh squeezed lemon juice
2 tbsp. corn oil
2 tbsp. butter
4 tbsp. GF soy sauce
salt to taste

Melt butter with corn oil on high heat in a large pot. Add rice, vegetables, soy sauce, and lemon juice. Fry on medium heat, stirring constantly, until browning develops. Scrape mixture to one side of pot, then scramble the two eggs on the opposite side. Once soft scrambled, incorporate with rice. Salt to taste, and add additional GF soy sauce, if desired. Once rice is fried and ready, add boiled shrimp. Stir just long enough for shrimp to heat in mixture, then remove from heat; do not overcook shrimp.

Recipe Contributor: Lauren Hatfield

mexican lasagna

2 large cans old el paso brand mild enchilada sauce
white corn tortillas (most brands are gf, but confirm they don't have flour or other gluten ingredients slipped in)
8-12oz. shredded sharp cheddar cheese
8-12oz. shredded pepper jack cheese
(optional) 1 lb ground beef
(optional) taco seasoning packet

Super quick & easy recipe for a busy night! If you like meat, brown your ground beef and cook in the taco seasoning as instructed on the packet. Next, use a 9x12 casserole dish, and spread a bit of the sauce on the bottom. Place a layer of tortillas next – I use 4-5 of them (the ones I use are about 6" in diameter), and tear as needed to piece in the holes. Then drizzle more sauce over them (I evenly spread it onto the tortillas with a spoon, but that might just be an OCD thing). Next, sprinkle a layer of the ground beef, and then sprinkle a generous layer of cheddar cheese. Start your layering over again with more tortillas, sauce, beef, and then the pepper jack. Repeat until your dish is decently full, and finish it off with sauce and then cheese. I tend to be heavy-handed with the sauce since the tortillas are often quite dry. Any excess sauce from the dish is great as a "gravy" for your rice. Pair with the mexican rice & beans recipe for a great dinner. Bake at 350 degrees for 20 minutes.

Recipe Contributor: Lauren Hatfield

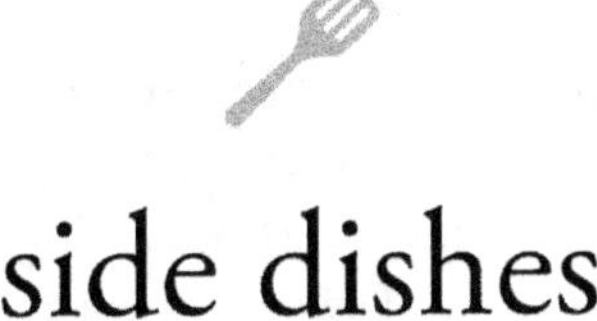

side dishes

parmesan seasoned new potatoes

1 bag fresh baby potatoes
1 bag fresh baby red potatoes (optional)
1 tbsp. olive oil (roughly)
1/2 - 1 c. parmesan cheese
2 tbsp. italian seasoning
1 tsp. garlic powder
1 tsp. onion salt
1 tsp. seasoned salt
salt & pepper to taste

This recipe is super easy! I'm sorry I can't be more specific with some of my amounts, but sometimes you need to channel your chef instincts with seasonings. This one is tough to mess up, so feel free to just sprinkle as you see fit on each seasoning. Cut baby potatoes into quarters. I include the second bag (red potatoes) if I'm cooking for a larger party. Place in a baking dish and drizzle with olive oil – just enough to barely moisten- and toss well. Add the rest of your seasonings and toss well again prior to baking. I recommend covering with foil and depressing the corners a bit to keep moisture inside.

Bake at 375 degrees for 45 minutes – 1 hour or until potatoes are well cooked.

Recipe Contributor: Lauren Hatfield

squash casserole

2 lbs. yellow squash, sliced
1 onion, finely chopped
1 tsp. salt
3 tbsp. butter, melted
3 tbsp. GF flour
2 eggs, slightly beaten
1 c. milk
16 oz. sharp cheddar cheese, grated
buttered GF breadcrumbs (or well crushed GF crackers)

Simmer squash and onions until tender, in about 1 inch of salted water with tight fitting lid (roughly 20 minutes). Drain well & mash (might need to drain a little more after mashing). Add other ingredients and pour into baking dish. Top with the buttered bread crumbs.

Bake at 350 degrees for 30-40 minutes

Recipe Contributor: Rosemary Watts
GF Adaptations: Lauren Hatfield

thanksgiving stuffing/dressing

4 c. GF breadcrumbs (dried Udi's bread in food processor)
2 c. GF cornbread crumbs (Bob's Red Mill makes a great cornbread mix for this)
4 tbsp. melted butter
1/2 c. chopped celery
2 tbsp. chopped onion
salt & pepper to taste
2 tbsp. sage
chicken broth to moisten

Mix all ingredients except broth. Add only enough broth to lightly moisten.

Bake at 375 for about 40 minutes to 1 hour, or until golden brown

Recipe Contributor: Margaret Watts
GF Adaptations: Lauren Hatfield

sweet potato soufflé

3 c. cooked sweet potato
1/2c. – 1 c. sugar
2 eggs, slightly beaten
1/2 c. milk
1/4 tsp. salt
1/3 c. butter, melted
1/2 tsp. vanilla

Topping:
1 c. brown sugar
1/3 c. melted butter
1/4 c. GF flour
1/2 c. chopped pecans

So delicious, it could easily pass for dessert! Mix ingredients with fork or mixer until smooth; put in casserole dish. Combine topping ingredients and evenly crumble over top.

Bake at 350 degrees for 30-40 minutes

Recipe Contributor: Rosemary Watts
GF Adaptations: Lauren Hatfield

mixed vegetable casserole

1 bag frozen mixed vegetables
1 onion, finely chopped
1/2 c. – 1 c. mayonnaise
2 c. sharp cheddar cheese, grated
buttered GF breadcrumbs (or well crushed GF crackers)

Cook mixed vegetables according to package instructions and drain well. Mix with remaining ingredients and pour into casserole dish. Top with buttered GF breadcrumbs.

Bake at 350 degrees for 30-40 minutes

Recipe Contributor: Rosemary Watts
GF Adaptations: Lauren Hatfield

cheesy grits soufflé

1 c. white grits (not instant)
2 tsp. salt
1 1/2 c. sharp cheddar cheese, grated
1 c. half and half
2 c. homemade chicken stock + 1 c. water
1 tbsp. minced garlic
5 eggs, separated
4 tbsp. unsalted butter
1/2 c. green onion, well chopped
ground black pepper and hot sauce to taste

In a large saucepan, boil the stock, half and half, water, and salt. Stir in the grits, and reduce to medium heat. Continue to cook, stirring often, until thick and creamy. Beat egg yolks, and temper with one spoonful of hot grits (continuing to stir). Add yolk mixture into hot grits. Add cheese, garlic, butter, and optional seasonings; stir well. An hour before serving, beat egg whites in a stainless steel bowl until they form stiff peaks. Gently fold the egg whites into your grits mixture and spoon into buttered baking dish.

Bake at 375 degrees for 30-40 minutes until the grits are set. Serve immediately.

Recipe: *Not Afraid of Flavor: Recipes from Magnolia Grill*
by Ben & Karen Barker, UNC Press ISBN 978-0-8078-5498-3
Published: September 2003

cheesy baked macaroni

3 eggs, slightly beaten
8 oz. GF macaroni
roughly 20 GF crackers (I recommend a half box of
Glutino's Table Crackers – NOT their round crackers)
salt to taste
milk to thin
1 tbsp. melted butter
16 oz. sharp cheddar cheese, grated

Cook macaroni according to package instructions, draining well. Crush crackers, and combine all ingredients (be careful to temper eggs around hot noodles or butter).

Bake at 350 degrees for 30-45 minutes, or until slightly golden.

Recipe Contributor: Margaret Watts
GF Adaptations: Lauren Hatfield

broccoli casserole

2 packages frozen chopped broccoli
1 can GF cream of mushroom soup
2 eggs, slightly beaten
1 onion, finely chopped
1/2 c. mayonnaise
2 c. sharp cheddar cheese, grated

Cook broccoli according to package instructions and drain well. Mix ingredients, being careful to temper eggs.

Bake at 350 degrees for 30 minutes

Recipe Contributor: Rosemary Watts
GF Adaptations: Lauren Hatfield

pineapple casserole

2 1lb.4oz. cans chunked pineapple, drained
2/3 c. sugar
2c. shredded sharp cheddar cheese
6 tbsp. GF flour (I recommend Pamela's cup for cup or
Pamela's baking and pancake mix)
1/2 package Glutino table crackers (not round crackers)
1 stick butter, melted

I fully recognize that mixing pineapple and cheese sounds incredibly strange. But it tastes fantastic, trust me! Combine pineapple, GF flour, sugar, & cheese. Pour in baking dish. Crush crackers and blend with margarine (works well in food processor); sprinkle on top of dish.

Bake at 350 degrees for 15 minutes

Recipe Contributor: Rosemary Watts
GF Adaptations: Lauren Hatfield

cranberry jell-o salad

1 can cranberries (sauce or whole berry)
1 c. boiling water
1 small can crushed pineapple
1 orange, chopped
1 large box of cherry jell-o
1/2 c. chopped pecans (optional)

Dissolve jell-o and cranberry sauce with boiling water. Add other ingredients and chill well until set.

Recipe Contributor: Rosemary Watts
GF Adaptations: Lauren Hatfield

lime jell-o salad

1 large package of lime jell-o
1 c. boiling water
1 1/2 c. cold water
3 oz. package of cream cheese, softened
2 cubed oranges
9 1/2 oz. can crushed pineapple, including juice
1 c. fruit cocktail, drained

Dissolve jell-o in boiling water. Add cold water. Beat cream cheese into mixture well. Add pineapple & other ingredients. Chill well until firm.

Recipe Contributor: Margaret Watts

carrot salad

3 c. shredded carrots
1/2 c. flaked coconut
1/2 c. raisins (or more!)
1/3 c. mayonnaise
1/4 c. pineapple juice
1/3 c. cashews

Mix all ingredients well. Chill 2-3 hours.

Recipe Contributor: Marilyn Doolittle

mexican rice & beans

2 c. rice (any rice you prefer. we use jasmine rice)
4 c. water (unless your rice has different water ratios for cooking)
5 tbsp. butter
1 packet of Goya brand seasoning - the one with saffron
1 tsp. onion salt
1 tsp. salt (more or less, depending on your taste)
1 tsp. dried cilantro
2 tsp. hot sauce of your choice
1-2 cans of light red kidney beans

Combine all ingredients (except beans) in a pot with a tight fitting lid. Bring to a boil on high heat. Once boiling, give mixture a quick stir and turn to low heat, placing the lid on the pot. Allow to simmer on low for 20 minutes, then remove from heat to sit another 10 minutes. Be sure to keep the lid on throughout the entire 30 minutes so the rice may properly steam. Then drain kidney beans and stir into your rice. Adjust salt as needed.

Recipe Contributor: Lauren Hatfield

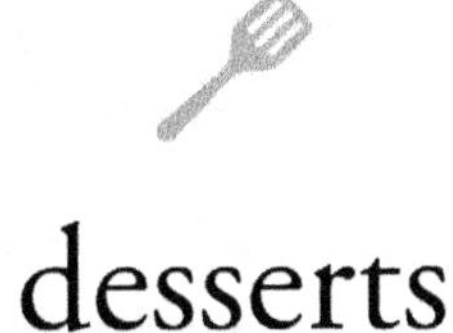

desserts

angel food cake

1 c. pamela's baking mix
1 ½ c. sugar
12 egg whites (or substitute)
1 ½ tsp. gf vanilla extract
1 ½ tsp. cream of tartar
½ tsp. salt

Preheat oven to 375. Be sure your 10" tube pan is clean & dry (any oil or residue can deflate egg whites). Sift together baking mix & 3/4c. of the sugar and set aside. In large bowl, whip the egg whites with the vanilla, cream of tartar, and salt to stiff peaks. Gradually add remaining sugar while continuing to whip to stiff peaks. When mixture is at maximum volume, fold in sifted ingredients gradually, 1/3 at a time. Do not over mix! Put the batter in the tube pan & bake 40-45 minutes until cake springs back. When cool, run a knife around the edge of the pan and invert.

Bake at 375 degrees for 40-45 minutes

Recipe Contributor: Lauren Hatfield

strawberry cobbler

2c. fresh fruit, well drained (I use strawberries - they're my favorite!) Frozen fruit often adds too much liquid
1 stick melted butter (1/2c.)
1 ½ c. Pamela's Baking mix
¾ c. milk
1 c. sugar

Melt butter in bottom of a 8"x 8" or 9"x 9" baking dish. In a separate bowl, combine baking mix, sugar, and milk. Evenly pour (plop, really) this mixture over the butter. Then scatter fruit over the top (might need to LIGHTLY mix a bit with a fork so some fruit goes toward the bottom). Bake 45 minutes to an hour. I would say until golden, but gluten free items like to stay undercooked in the middle. So I cook it until it doesn't juggle in the middle too much anymore without the top burning.

Bake at 350 degrees for 45 – 60 minutes.

Recipe Contributor: Rosemary Watts
GF Adaptations: Lauren Hatfield

pumpkin pie

2 c. pumpkin (canned or fresh)
2 eggs
1 tbsp. Pamela's baking mix
½ tsp. salt (optional)
1 c. sugar
1-1 ½ tsp pumpkin pie spice
7 oz. evaporated milk

Mix all ingredients well. Prep pie shells according to their instructions. Pour into pie shell(s) about 3/4 full (makes two pies for small crusts). I use the Whole Foods Gluten Free Bakehouse shells, and I usually double the recipe which leaves some filling leftover. I like to bake that in little ramekins for a treat later on. Bake the pies until the center is solidified when wiggled - that's my sophisticated explanation.

Bake at 325 degrees for 1 hour

Recipe Contributor: Margaret Watts
GF Adaptations: Lauren Hatfield

peppermint snowball truffles

1 ½ packs GF Oreo-style cookies (or 1 pack of regular)
8 oz. cream cheese, softened
dash of peppermint extract
white chocolate chips
crushed candy canes

Crumble cookies in food processor. Add 8oz. cream cheese and peppermint extract; mix well. Roll into 1" – 1 ½" balls & put on cookie sheet (line bottom with parchment or wax paper). Sometimes I put a little nonstick spray or coconut oil on my hands before starting to keep the balls from sticking as I roll them. Freeze 30 minutes to 1 hr. Melt white chocolate chips according to package instructions. Roll/dip balls in white chocolate and sprinkle with crushed candy canes before chocolate solidifies. Serve once cooled; keep refrigerated.

Recipe Contributor: Alison Watts

oatmeal raisin cookies

20 tbsp. butter, softened
1 ½ c. Pamela's baking mix
¾ c. firmly packed brown sugar
½ c. granulated sugar
1 tsp. baking soda
1 ½ tsp. cinnamon
½ tsp. salt (optional)
2 eggs
1 tsp. gf vanilla
3 c. gluten free oats, uncooked
1 c. raisins

Beat both sugars and softened butter on medium speed until smooth. Add eggs and vanilla, continuing to beat well. Combine baking mix, baking soda, cinnamon, and salt separately; then add to mixture. Last, add raisins and oats, incorporating well. Place rounded tablespoons onto ungreased cookie sheets. Bake 8-10 minutes, or until just beginning to lightly brown. Cool for one minute on the sheet, then remove to wire rack to finish cooling. Store tightly covered.

Bake at 350 degrees for 8-10 minutes

Recipe Contributor: Lauren Hatfield

milkin' cookies (lactation)

1 c. sugar
1 c. brown sugar
1 c. butter
1 tsp vanilla
2 eggs
2 tbsp ground flaxseed in 4tbsp water (let this sit while you mix everything else)
2-4 tbsp nutritional yeast (GF)
1 tsp salt
1 tsp baking soda
2 c. gf all-purpose flour
3 c. old fashioned gluten free oats
1 c. chocolate chips

Optional add-ins - ½ c. peanut butter
For Grown-Up Girl Scouts add 1/2c finely shredded coconut and caramel chips.

Cream fats and sugar, add in eggs, vanilla, and flaxseed goo. Mix dry ingredients and add in, mix until blended. Stir in oats, and your chosen add-ins. For bars - bake at 350 degrees for 30min. For cookies, drop on a greased cookie sheet and bake for 12 minutes.

Recipe Source: Jamilla Walker, The Labor Ladies
GF Adaptations: Lauren Hatfield

no-bake "school" cookies

2 c. sugar
4 tbsp. cocoa
2 ½ c. quick-cook gluten free oats
1 stick butter (1/2 c.)
½ c. evaporated milk
1 tsp. gf vanilla
½ c. peanut butter

Boil sugar, butter, milk, cocoa 1 minute, stirring constantly. Remove from heat. Add the rest of the ingredients, working quickly. Drop by rounded spoonfuls onto wax paper or parchment. Allow to cool at room temperature

Recipe Contributor: Rosemary Watts
GF Adaptations: Lauren Hatfield

gooey cake

1 package yellow gf cake mix (be sure it's a brand that yields a full cake…such as Namaste. Many only yield a half cake. Otherwise, use 2 packages)
1 stick butter (1/2 c.)
1 egg

Mix ingredients and pat into ungreased 9" x 13" pan. Then add second layer:

1 block of cream cheese, softened
2 eggs
1lb box of confectioner's sugar
1 tsp. vanilla

Cream ingredients together and spread over first layer.

Bake at 350 degrees for 35 minutes, or until golden brown

Recipe Contributor: Lauren Hatfield

million dollar pie

1 can sweetened condensed milk
¼ c. lemon juice
½ c. chopped pecans
½ c. coconut
1 small can crushed pineapple, drained
1 large container of whipped cream
2 gluten free pie shells

Bake pie shells completely according to their instructions & allow to cool at room temperature. Combine ingredients and fill shells. Chill at least 4 hours.

Recipe Contributor: Margaret Watts
GF Adaptations: Lauren Hatfield

simple cheesecake

crust:
1 ½ c. gf graham cracker or ginger snap crumbs
¼ c. confectioners' sugar
1/3 c. melted butter
mix & press into bottom and sides of a 9" pan (or adapt for a spring form pan)

filling:
2 c. (2 large packages) cream cheese, softened
2 eggs
2/3 c. sugar
1 tsp. gf vanilla extract

Beat on medium speed until smooth. Fill crust and bake on cookie sheet (to prevent burning crust base) for 20 minutes. Add crust shield (or foil) and bake an additional 10-20 minutes, or until just starting to golden. Cool on rack and then refrigerate once cool.

Bake at 350 degrees for 20 minutes + 10-20

Recipe Contributor: Lauren Hatfield

chocolate cherry cookies

1 ½ c. pamela's baking mix or other gf flour
½ c. cocoa
¼ tsp. baking powder
¼ tsp. salt
¼ tsp. baking soda
1 stick butter, softened
1 c. sugar
1 egg
1 ½ tsp. vanilla

frosting:
10oz jar maraschino cherries (reserve juice)
6 oz package semi-sweet chocolate chips
½ c. sweetened condensed milk

Mix dry ingredients together. In a large mixing bowl, beat butter and sugar until fluffy. Add egg and vanilla; beat well. Add dry ingredients to creamed mixture and mix until well blended (dough will be quite stiff). Shape dough into 35 1" balls and place on ungreased cookie sheet. Press your thumb into the center of each ball and place a cherry in the print. In a sauce pan, combine sweetened condensed milk and chocolate chips; heat just until melted. Add 4 tsp. cherry juice (stir), and spoon frosting over each cookie. Bake at 350 degrees for 10 minutes; remove from pan with spatula and place on cooling rack.

Recipe Contributor: Marilyn Doolittle

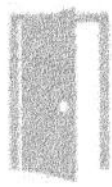

coming out of the pantry

In closing this book, I've asked my fellow celiacs or gluten-challenged friends to air their dirty laundry, sharing stories from their own experiences. Some stories have fabricated names to protect privacy. Everyone's gluteny past has something to learn, and hopefully you'll see you aren't alone. Thank you to these dear friends. Enjoy!

jessica paulsen

"For years - almost a decade of my life - I lived with spasms of abdominal pain that eventually took over my life. The issue of gluten sensitivity, for me, is that it crept up slowly. I didn't just wake up one morning in horrid pain. Instead, I would have random occurrences of extreme pain and cramping but then things would settle down. It wasn't until I was pregnant with my son that I began to realize that something wasn't right with how my body was digesting food.

When my OB asked if I had felt any Braxton Hicks contractions, all I could answer was that my stomach felt like I was having contractions constantly and it had been that way for years. So I became pretty nervous that I would not know when labor actually arrived, and that is what happened. I was 5cm dilated without realizing I was in labor, because the pain felt like the pain that occurred every day. I wish I had given up gluten then, but no, I'm pretty stubborn. I came up with a list of other foods to avoid, but give up gluten? No, way!

Fast forward a few years and I was instructing my 3 year old son on how to call 911 if Mama passed out in the bathroom because that is what I thought would eventually happen. The final straw was when I began using breathing techniques for labor pains to get through the abdominal cramping numerous times a day. I then accepted the fact that I couldn't ignore this any longer.

Within a month of being gluten free, I could tell a vast difference. Not only was my pain absent, but also my energy level soared and my irritability almost vanished.

I have now (2015) been gluten free for 3 1/2 years and egg free for 2 1/2 years. Looking back at all the years and the time spent in bathrooms with agonizing pain, I can't believe it took me so long to make the change. Initially, it was very frustrating to cut out so much of my favorite food and have to read labels on every single item I bought. But eventually, it becomes a way of life and you'll never want to go back.

The pain isn't worth it!"

visit jessica's great recipes and advice at:
www.thelocalgoodness.com

maryann thompson

"Hello, all! My gluten story is probably rather boring, compared to most. I didn't show symptoms until I was in my thirties, and even then, they didn't arrive with fireworks.

Every holiday meal since I was young, I remembered my grandfather complaining that he didn't like my mom's cooking. He loved the taste, but said that every time he ate there, he would go home with a stomachache. We all thought he was just being his grumpy old man self that couldn't be pleased. He wasn't the type to go to a doctor, either, so we wrote it off. Stay with me, I promise there's a point coming.

Once I received my first big promotion at age 32, I began to notice a trend of mild nausea after each meal. I suppose I noticed it more because the new position brought much travel (which also meant much dining out and take out)! I was eating antacids like they were candy, and also noticed how exhausted I became. I would count down the hours each day until I could crash in my hotel room – what a drag! I never got to enjoy the scenery in all the lovely places I was traveling because I was too tired.

It was one fateful Thanksgiving, when I was home enjoying our feast, that I slumped on the sofa after dinner with a grunt. "Mommmmm, where do you keep your antacids these days?" I moaned. She said, "You know, you sound an awful lot like Grandpa Frank, Lizzy."

That's when it hit me. Grandpa Frank ate all his meals at his home – he never left the house except to come to Mom's for holidays. His home diet consisted mostly of canned vegetables and frozen meats that he ordered to his doorstep for thawing and popping in the oven. Mom's foods were heavily breaded southern dishes with lots of rolls and desserts. No wonder the man thought her food made him sick – it actually did! This just couldn't be a coincidence, and I must not have fallen too far from that grouchy old tree.

I'm sure you've guessed the rest of my story. A trip to the doctor introduced me to gluten and how it could be affecting me. Strangely, though, I tested negative for celiac disease.

There are many studies out now saying gluten sensitivity doesn't exist, but my stomach (and doctors) say differently. I've been able to enjoy life again since kicking the gluten. I have energy for miles and can actually see all those beautiful cities when I travel! No more purchasing antacid in bulk, and no more nausea. I have never felt better in my life, and I owe it to a gluten free diet. I don't know the science, but I know that my body was extremely responsive to gluten.

How did things turn out with Grandpa Frank? Well, he won't listen to reason and just keeps eating/complaining each holiday. He secretly loves the food too much to quit, but I didn't tell you that."

elizabeth johnson

"Hi! My name is Elizabeth and I'm 23 years old. I live in Canada and I have celiac disease. I was diagnosed about three years ago now, but I remember being fifteen when the symptoms started. I was suddenly sick all the time, but I had no idea why. My immunity was terrible; I almost always had a cold. I was also always bloated and I remember thinking to myself, "One day this will mean something - this isn't normal!"

For years, I watched my health slowly deteriorate. I was getting so tired that I had to take naps every day. I rarely left the house other than to go to school. I had constant nausea and brain fog. It progressed to the point where I was vomiting constantly for months (gross, I know).

After six years of doctor visits and being told all my symptoms were from stress, I was finally given a diagnosis – celiac disease. "This will be easy," I thought. "I'll just cut out bread and start feeling normal." Boy, was I wrong!

It has taken me years to completely figure out the gluten free diet. I still make mistakes sometimes. It's so easy to slip up. I have stopped eating out (which isn't for everyone) and no longer eat gluten free processed foods, which has helped. It's been a long road but it has all made me a better person - I appreciate life a lot more then I used to! I really enjoy cooking all my own meals; it keeps me on track with being healthy. There are so many delicious naturally gluten free recipes now, which made changing my diet so much easier! It was a slow recovery, but I'm thankful I received a diagnosis and can now live a life free of all those health problems."

sophie anderson

"I'm a bit embarrassed that I am writing such personal things here, but I also know that the people reading might be as desperate as I was. While the comings and goings of my bathroom habits aren't exactly glamorous, neither are yours...which means you don't get to judge me. Haha!

I was diagnosed at a super young age with IBS. Doctors weren't as familiar with celiac disease back then, but I've heard it is most often diagnosed in children these days. Praise God these little ones get the opportunity I didn't!

The doctor recommended all sorts of treatments (including diet changes, though not gluten), but most of them didn't help much. Life in one's formative years are always difficult, trying to fit in and whatnot; add in unpredictable diarrhea, and I quickly had some heartbreaking moments that no child should endure.

I at least knew that dairy was a trigger, which helped lessen the situation some. My poor mom didn't know what else to do, so to survive it all, she simply gave me a dose of over-the-counter diarrhea medicine each morning. I certainly don't recommend that as a long-term solution (nor do most doctors), but it at least allowed me to go to school without constant fear of an embarrassing situation.

Fast-forward to my first year of college, which brought all new "fun." In the first few months, I made some immature decisions (hey, we all did – don't lie!), and I found myself consuming a little bit more alcohol than I should have. This multiplied my situation, causing a few relived memories I hoped I'd never see again.

Luckily, the university I attended was in a bigger and more progressive city than the one in which I was raised. When I explained my story to the health facility doctor on campus, she was on point! Her first suggestion was the simple blood test for celiac disease; within days, it was confirmed!

I ended up doing as much research on gluten as I was doing for my other assignments. As I learned what I could/couldn't eat, the dining hall became a difficult hurdle, as well. The employees didn't enjoy their jobs at this particular campus, and certainly didn't have the patience to accommodate a difficult order. This prompted me to sharpen my cooking skills, even in the confines of a dorm room. You should see what I can do with a hot plate!

So today, I am finally able to enjoy eating. It was a long road for me, and my entire childhood made me believe this was just the way I was – the way life would always be. I'm so thankful for that campus doctor's knowledge and quick response!

And hey, at least I was able to dodge the "freshman fifteen" before it even happened!"

sarah miller

"Growing up, I was the kid with terrible acne. My acne was so relentless that it created some pretty severe scarring. As I reached age seventeen, it had mostly cleared up…much to the joy of my self-conscious teenage self!

But as each year passed, new skin conditions developed. There were bumpy, scaly patches at my elbows, neck, and knees all throughout college. Some days they would peel and bleed, causing them to appear even worse (because they were so itchy and I scratched constantly). Some doctors called it eczema, while others said it could be psoriasis. They suggested that since I had acne, I was just "one of those people prone to skin trouble." I used every cream on the market, including steroids, antibiotics, and even homeopathic remedies/oils.

Years later, I tried a new dermatologist when I moved to a new city. He performed further tests, many of which were as inconclusive as those from years past. It was his (brilliant!) idea to try cutting out gluten. First of all, I had only heard the word "gluten" from my hippie friends, and I assumed it was something they made up as a diet fad. Upon further explanation, the doctor warned that giving this up might be difficult, but we should at least try it for a month. I had tried everything else, so what did I have to lose?

To my surprise, it worked! Well, mostly. I still have mild

spots here and there, but I'd say about 90% of it is GONE! Apparently, celiac disease (which was a confirmed diagnosis later) can present as a skin reaction called dermatitis herpetiformis. I was thrilled to finally be free! And to think, I could've avoided all those costly and dangerous medications for years if only I changed my food."

cara hasco

Hello, all! Just to give you a bit of background information, those closest to me are aware of my deep love for children. Well, at least that's the way it is *now*...

You see, as a youth, I always assumed I'd have the expected 2 babies when I grew up (one boy and one girl, naturally). I was in a family with two children, and most everyone I knew was in a family with two children. Therefore, it was destiny and not much of a thought otherwise.

As I grew into my spunky high school years, life became defined by social events. I attended every football game to support my friends, the girls had a movie night every Tuesday, and the weekends were spent at friends' houses or parties. This social calendar was also about to change in a big way one September evening.

The Friday night football game had just finished, so several of us went to grab pizza. Halfway through the meal, a stabbing pain doubled me over into the floor; I was in the most wretched agony I've ever experienced. That room full of 16 year olds went into full panic mode, calling 911 and my parents. My family arrived at the hospital shortly after the ambulance, but they hardly recognized my colorless face. I was numb with fear.

After what seemed like endless hours of testing, the pain gradually weakened to a dull ache. The hospital had no results, and sent me away with prescription strength ibuprofen and recommendations on gastrointestinal specialists for follow-up.

I began rigorous testing on a variety of gastrointestinal disorders. Throughout the process, I had a very restricted diet to minimize distress to my intestines. Naturally, this made a high schooler's social occasions quite a bit more difficult. I became a recluse, wading in a pool of growing depression at home. The tests were not yielding results, and I had little motivation to even complete schoolwork each day.

Concerned about the direction things were heading, my doctor recommended I begin an anti-depressant medication, as well as setting up appointments with a counselor.

That only made things worse. The first counselor I visited told me chronic illness is a very specialized form of counseling for which she was not qualified. She said her best suggestion was that I get a plant, and then she took my parents' money for the session. The second counselor simply wanted to increase my medications, which only worsened my gastrointestinal upset. At this point, it was a cycle and my pain only became worse.

Finally, during one of many colonoscopies, my doctors found a spot they hadn't been able to detect in all their other studies. I was quickly diagnosed with Chrohn's disease, and rushed into surgery to remove the enflamed tissue.

I healed quickly, and we adjusted my diet accordingly. We noticed a strong correlation between my flare-ups and gluten. Once I went gluten and lactose free, little flashes of color finally returned to my face (and my spirit). Though I was doing better, I still had symptoms on a day to day basis. My body responded to standard treatments, but only to a certain point.

So, what does this story have to do with my love of children?

You see, after many of life's milestones whizzed by over the years, I found myself with a wonderful husband and newly pregnant. I also found myself horribly nauseous, with a condition called Hyperemesis Gravidarum. It's basically morning sickness times a thousand.

One rainy day, as I was finally approaching my second trimester and emerging from the fog, I lifted my dizzy head from the pillow with a startling realization: my intestines felt great. Not one day in the decades between high school and that day had I ever experienced a day without (at the very least) slight cramping. All the nausea kept me distracted for the months this intestinal change had been taking place. But that fateful day, I was elated with my discovery.

To my surprise, not only did my nausea subside for the balance of the pregnancy, but my intestines worked like a charm. This continued until I finished breastfeeding, when I began to notice my old symptoms returning.

So, what does one do when pregnancy is the only solution to a tricky medical problem? One prepares herself for the idea of a big family in her future!

I'm mostly joking about that (I began wishing for a bigger family throughout college, anyway), but I can't deny the correlation. It was so nice to finally have moments free of my chains, even if it was during other pregnancy symptoms.

I'm now the proud mom of 6 children, with one on the way. We are excited to have the privilege of raising this family, and I have enjoyed every step of the journey.

---

about the author

Lauren Hatfield is a wife, mom of three, designer, model, and most importantly – a daughter of the King. For more than a decade, Lauren's professional career has focused on marketing and design, with specialties including graphic design, web design, product design, and more.

After battling chronic illness since 2007 with some of the best doctors in the world, Lauren's journey still hasn't produced a solid diagnosis or completely successful treatment plan. She seeks to use her story to encourage and inform others who are walking a similar path.

Lauren owns a design business called Valentia Ifuerza, a derivative of the Spanish for "courage and strength." VI is a fashion & product line that promotes wellness through a variety of handmade items, including custom/couture veils, Italian leather handbags, decadent aromatherapy spa products, jewelry, and so much more.

A portion of every VI sale is donated to celiac disease research, and a portion of every veil sale supports those with special needs.

Please visit the website: vi-style.com

www.ingramcontent.com/pod-product-compliance
Lightning Source LLC
Chambersburg PA
CBHW070231210526
45168CB00020B/1888

9781506129006